House Dust Mite

~ a partnership for life

Dr Stephen J Connellan

Copyright © 2015 Dr S J Connellan

All rights reserved

ISBN: 1495241106
ISBN-13: 978-1495241109

DEDICATION

To all those sufferers who are forced to co-habit with this mite.

CONTENTS

Graphics by Dr Connellan

1	An introduction to the House Dust Mite	8
2	The mechanism of mite allergy	13
3	Can we make life more difficult for mites?	16
4	Treatment	18
5	Research	20
6	References	26

ACKNOWLEDGEMENTS

With thanks to all of the expert opinion provided by organisations and specialist societies that continue to publish valuable peer reviewed conclusions that help us to plan management strategies in healthcare.

Chapter 1

AN INTRODUCTION TO THE HOUSE DUST MITE

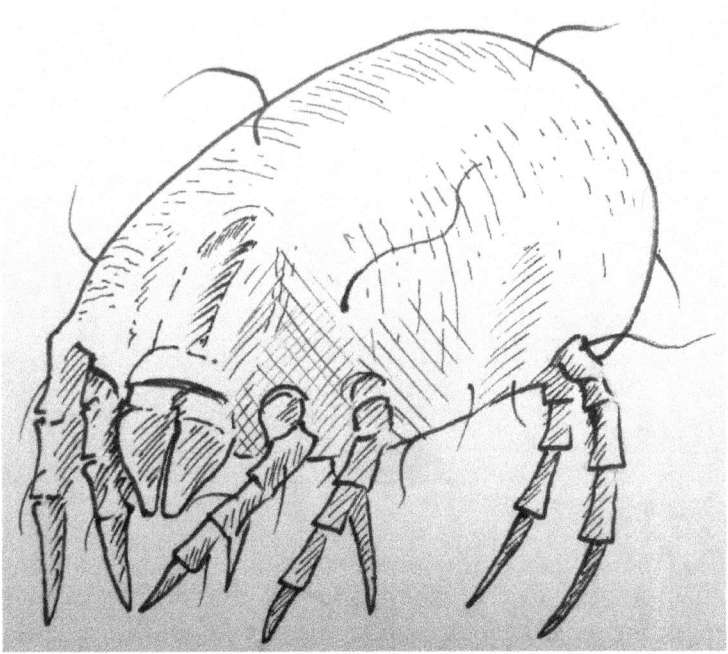

HISTORY AND EVOLUTION

Why would you bother to read a book about a tiny creature which is not even visible to the naked eye? Whether you like it or not, it has become a life time partner for the majority of the planet's house dwelling population and its life is intimately linked with ours. If we think of our dwelling as a nest then we share it with this tiny partner and it relies on us for its food, shelter, warmth and 'drink'.

If we consider that some estimates reckon that the house dust mite (referred to as 'the mite' from now on) has been active on earth for around 20 million years, then it would not be unreasonable to consider the human race as a much more recent species which is being used by the mite.

Perhaps our species will eventually become extinct and the mite will move on to some alternative host!

In a remarkable study by Klimov and O'Connor [1], they concluded that the very earliest free-living mites (related to spiders as they have 8 legs) evolved in to parasites in the nests of warm-blooded animals but then further adapted to become free-living again. It had always been postulated that when a creature evolved to a particular more specialised existence, it would not return to an earlier pattern of living. This latest free-living existence enabled the mite to migrate to human dwellings where it has thrived ever since.

The crucial adaptations included tolerance of lower humidity and most importantly the development of powerful digestive enzymes. These allowed them to feed on keratin (skin scales, hair, feathers and finger nails). They became much less dependent on specific hosts and were happy to stay with any that could provide the necessary 'home comforts'.

The 'fancy' name for the European variant of the mite is Dermatophagoides Pteronyssinus and is derived from the Greek and literally means 'skin eating feather loving'. The North American variant of the mite is Dermatophagoides Farinae and the latter word is based on the Latin for flour due to its preferred habitat. There are, in fact, more than 700 mite species!

BODY IMAGE

How would we recognize the mite if we bumped into it? Fortunately, in some ways, it is not possible to see them with the naked eye. The fact that our dwellings are teeming with them would tend to spook us out otherwise! You would need a 10 x magnifying glass to see them as they are about 0.01 inches long. To make it more difficult they are translucent. They have 8 hairy legs being related to spiders and also have hairs on their undersides. They don't have eyes or antennae and there are mouth parts at the front. The shell of the body is tough even though it is translucent. There is plenty of video footage of 'herds' of mites grazing away on skin scales. Just enter 'house dust mite' in a search on YouTube.

REPRODUCTION

After the adult female has laid around 60 eggs, each egg goes through a larval and then nymphal stage, finally emerging as an adult around one month later. Each adult will then live between 1 - 3 months which gives the females plenty of time to procreate. A mattress may house anything between 100,000 to 10 million mites depending on the bedroom environment and age of the mattress.

FOOD AND DRINK

As already mentioned, their primary food source is dander (skin scales) from humans and animals. In addition, they may consume debris which is keratinous, such as finger nails and feathers. However, they have a very eclectic diet which may include mouldy bread crumbs, pet food, cereals, fish food flakes, etc. As with most of us on this earth, water is essential for life and mites don't drink as such. They absorb water through their outer cuticle from the surrounding air. It is this fact that makes them vulnerable if the humidity is below 60%. They thrive when the relative humidity is around 75-80%. They also need a warm environment which would ideally be around 75 – 80 degrees F (24 – 27 degrees C).

Western civilization has been very kind to the mite. We stick on the central heating when it is cold outside, close all the double-glazed windows, affording little ventilation, dry wet clothes on the radiator, use gas appliances which increase ambient water vapour and even use an electric blanket to warm the bed. Our hospitality has ensured that the mite is well catered for. The highest mite densities occur in the summer months particularly when it is humid and conversely the lowest densities are in the drier winter periods, unless the home owner reproduces the warm humid conditions! They are usually absent in very arid climates. There will be transient higher ambient levels of mites during household chores such as bed making and vacuuming. In fact the less efficient vacuum cleaners will actually distribute the dust from under carpets up in to the general environment.

HOUSE DUST COMPOSITION

House dust comprises tracked in soil and airborne particles from outside. The remainder is made up of dead skin from the animal inhabitants, carpet and furniture fibres, food waste (some of it mouldy), insect remains and of course mites, both dead and alive, along with their faecal pellets and cast skins. Mites are not all bad news because they are excellent scavengers. A number of components of house dust are consumed by the mite and it even recycles its own faecal droppings by consuming those as well!

FAECAL DROPPINGS – THE BAD NEWS

In order to evolve in to an independent free-living mite it developed the facility to digest keratin by producing a special digestive juice. This contains proteolytic enzymes (enzymes which break down protein into digestible components). These have scientific labels such as Der p 1, relating to the Pteronyssinus variant or Der f 1 relating to the Farinae variant (there are several of these allergens so far identified). These activated enzymes will be present in the droppings of the mite and unfortunately they are highly allergenic. This means that the protein makeup of these enzymes tend to stimulate those susceptible humans in to producing antibodies (immunoglobulin E or IgE) specifically against this component of the droppings. The mite droppings usually comprise 3 to 5 balls stuck together by mucous and wrapped in a membrane. When this is deposited it may get eaten by another mite, broken down by local moisture or just broken up by general disturbance. A large dropping might be as big as 0.0015 inches! However, much smaller particles may get airborne. This latter fact is important as such small airborne particles which are carrying the proteolytic enzymes may then be inhaled deeply in to the lungs of susceptible individuals. There is also evidence that certain fungi will be present on the mite and in its droppings, having passed through its gut. Aspergillus is one of the species identified. It isn't thought, however, that this fungus is responsible for the allergy to the mite. There are also a number of other potential triggers for an immune response which include mite and bacterial proteins, endotoxin (a by-product of bacterial activity) and chitin (the outer covering of the mite). These may enhance the allergic response to the mite enzyme.

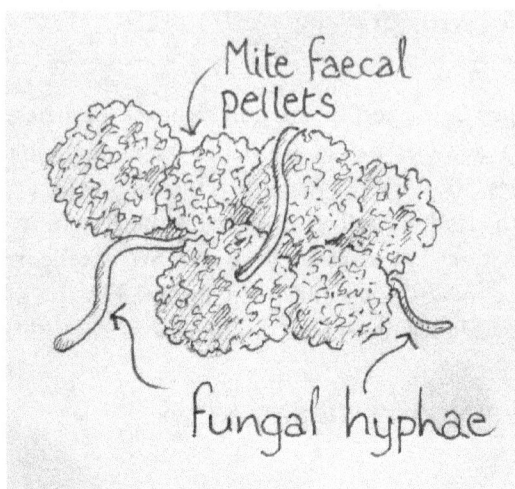

To complicate matters further it is now known that the mite enzymes can stimulate certain receptors on cells and cause them to react as they would to local inflammation. This is separate from an allergic reaction but it might make the inflamed mucosal linings more leaky and allow allergens and infections greater access to the underlying blood circulation.

Some of the protein in mite allergen (tropomysin) is similar in character to that seen in certain crustaceans and cockroaches and there is some evidence to suggest that allergy to mites could cross over to these other creatures. Some research has suggested that up to 15% of those highly sensitized to the mite are also sensitized to e.g. shrimps and snails. However, there is currently no evidence to suggest that such individuals should avoid eating shrimps (unless, of course, they have allergic symptoms closely correlated with eating them!).

Oral mite anaphylaxis (OMA or 'Pancake Syndrome') is a more recently recognized severe allergic reaction, which may result in anaphylaxis, following the ingestion of storage mite-contaminated wheat flour. The flour has usually been stored for months at ambient temperatures. The observed cases tend to be in warmer tropical environments, more often triggered by eating pancakes and with a history suggesting a tendency to allergic conditions, particularly mite but not wheat sensitivity.

Chapter 2

THE MECHANISM OF MITE ALLERGY

So what happens inside the susceptible individuals to result in this allergy to the mite. At some stage they must have inhaled some of the mite faecal material. Their immune system decided that this was a foreign protein which they needed protecting from (you can't always trust the human body to do the right thing!). It decided to produce a specific antibody which would latch on to the threatening protein if it should dare to invade again. This antibody is an immunoglobulin type E (IgE) which then searches the blood stream to find the mast cell which is also in the business of reacting to injuries and producing local inflammation. It is present in tissues which are exposed to the outside environment; e.g. nasal passage, airway, eyes, gut and skin. In this case the IgE is specifically targeted at Der p protein in the activated enzyme. When that protein entered their blood stream the next time, the specific IgE, now attached to the mast cell, latches on to the circulating enzyme protein and this causes the wall of the mast cell to break down and release all the histamine from the cell. The basophil is another circulating blood cell which will also be involved.

Exactly the same mechanism occurs in someone who has become allergic to grass pollen (one of the commonest forms of allergy). When the mast cell breaks down, the histamine and several other chemicals result in dilatation (widening) of blood vessels resulting in seepage of fluid in to the surrounding tissues. This results in congestion and swelling. The allergic individual will suffer nasal stuffiness, excess mucous (with sneezing), itchy nose/eyes and cough (due to the effect of histamine on local nerve supply). The airway smooth muscle may react by going into spasm causing the wheeze of asthma and excess mucous will be produced in the airways tending to make the airways even more narrowed. Other cells are 'recruited' to the area and they result in more prolonged inflammation.

The following graphic demonstrates the allergic process. In this case the allergen is pollen.

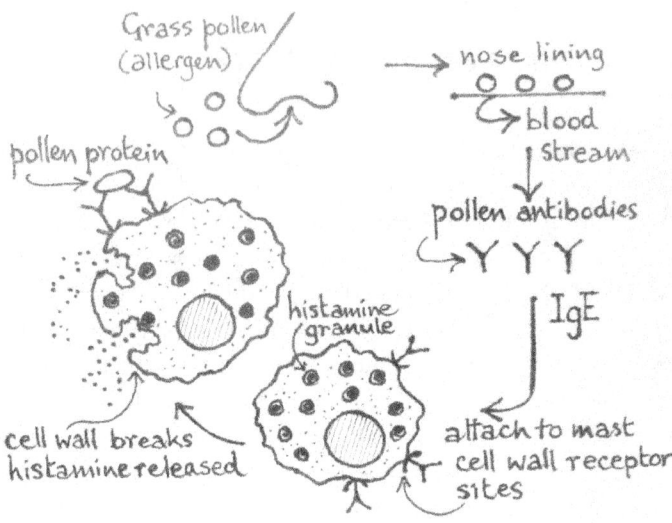

This is what a mast cell looks like under the microscope. The dark granules are stuffed with histamine.

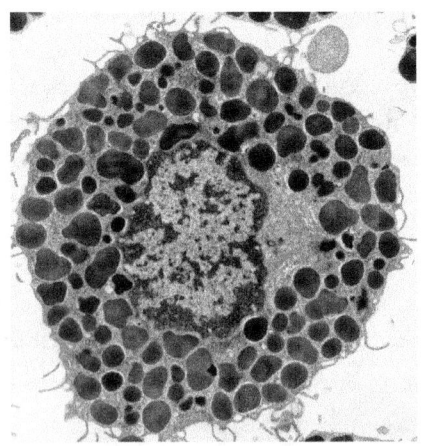

When first discovered by Paul Ehrlich in 1878 he thought the cell's role was to keep all the surrounding tissue well nourished. He must have felt that the granules were some form of sustenance. The German for 'fattening' is 'mast' and so his original name for them was 'mastzellen'.

Below is an example of an allergy skin test, demonstrating what is called a 'wheal and flare' reaction. The raised lump in the skin of the arm is at the site of a skin prick into a drop of fluid placed on the skin surface. Within the liquid is the protein or allergen responsible for the house dust mite sensitivity. The wheal is the visible raised lump and this can be measured to provide some estimate of the strength of reaction to the allergen. The flare is the darkened area around it (red if this picture was in colour!). This flushing is the result of the dilated blood vessels which have been stimulated by the local release of histamine. This gives us a beautifully graphic presentation of the underlying reaction that has occurred when the mite allergen has been delivered to the antibodies sitting on the wall of the mast cells, causing them to rupture and liberate histamine.

Now imagine that reaction occurring when many thousands of particles of tiny airborne mite faecal proteins are inhaled, land on the skin or get trapped in the linings of the nose or eyes.

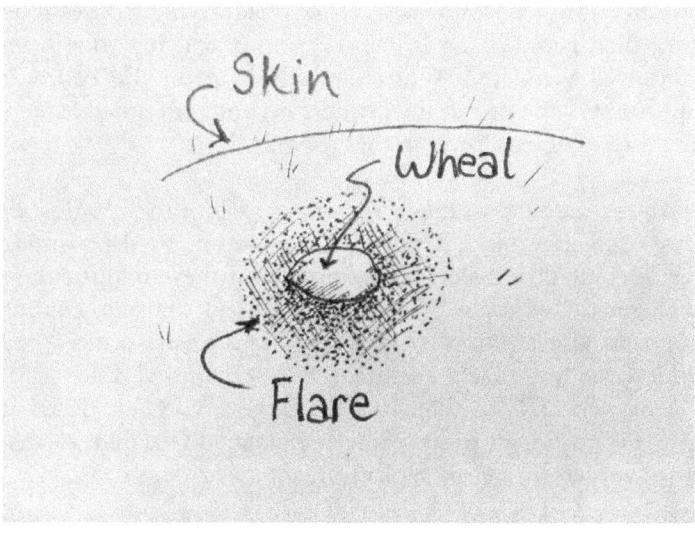

Chapter 3

CAN WE MAKE LIFE MORE DIFFICULT FOR MITES?

Most approaches aimed at reducing mite population are based on common sense and a full knowledge of the mite's preferences and lifestyle. However, it should be stated from the outset that anyone suffering with allergic reactions to mite droppings has the potential to react to tiny amounts of the allergen. It is also possible that they may be reacting to seasonal allergens and others in the home environment. This makes it very difficult to achieve complete resolution of symptoms in such individuals.

CAN WE REDUCE CONTACT WITH MITES?

We need to accept from the outset that it is very difficult to completely avoid all contact with mites. Living at high altitude with low humidity would reduce likely contact but isn't always an option!

As noted above the mites prefer warm and humid conditions and so it makes sense to keep kitchens and bathrooms well ventilated after bathing, washing and cooking. These rooms should be isolated from the rest of the accommodation at the times when their humidity is increased and windows and vents should be open whenever possible. The bottom line is to avoid any increase in damp environment. Try to avoid drying clothes indoors. If you have to, then avoid doing it in bedrooms and living rooms and keep those rooms well ventilated. When concentrating on the bedroom, take every opportunity to open the windows and if possible keep the temperature a few degrees lower in that room.

The clue is in the name 'dust mites' so it makes sense to keep dust down to a minimum – no easy task! Reduce all the clutter, books, soft toys and clothes that become dust collectors, particularly if they are difficult to clean. If you can't get rid of them then isolate them in drawers, cupboards or display cabinets. Use a damp cloth to regularly clean surfaces and don't forget window blinds which are great dust collectors! Use an efficient vacuum cleaner with HEPA filter to clean carpets, curtains, floors and soft furnishings. It is important to have a well maintained vacuum cleaner and a lot of house-workers forget to replace air filters or dust bags on a regular basis.

A poorly performing vacuum cleaner may just distribute the dust, accumulated under carpets, up in to the air.

Ideally, the mattress should also be vacuum-cleaned every fortnight. The washing machine temperature should be set at 60 degrees C for sheets, duvets and pillow cases and the wash repeated every 2 weeks. If possible, have curtains which can be washed at 60 degrees C as well. This temperature has been shown to kill mites. Duvets should be made of synthetic material and used preferably to blankets. Pillows, mattresses and duvets should be completely encased in micro-porous membrane covers which should be cleaned with a damp cloth whenever the bedding has been changed. Keep any stuffed toys to a minimum and put them in the freezer for 6 hours every month. Carpets are a significant problem so, wherever possible, replace with linoleum or have natural flooring such as wood or tiles. Failing that, synthetic carpets with short pile are best. Any rugs should be washable regularly at high temperatures. When buying any new furniture aim for canvas, cane or leather-covered which are much easier to clean and not a good surface for mites. A number of other products are on the market claiming to reduce mites. These include ionisers, air filters and dehumidifiers but, as yet, there aren't any definitive studies to confirm effectiveness.

Are dehumidifiers effective in reducing mite related symptoms?

A study by Custovic A et al [2] looked at the use of portable dehumidifiers in the control of house dust mites. Based on the principle that mites thrive in conditions of around 70% humidity, it would seem reasonable that reduction in humidity would reduce mite numbers. However, when 6 houses with and 6 houses without dehumidifiers were compared, there was no difference in mite counts in either of the groups, throughout the 3 month study. The conclusion was that a single portable dehumidifier placed centrally in a house is not capable of reducing overall indoor humidity to an effective level that would retard mite growth.

Are air filters effective in reducing mite related symptoms?

A review in Current Allergy and Asthma Reports by Sublett J L [3] looked at the effectiveness of air filters and air cleaners in allergic respiratory disease. A summary of their conclusions is outlined in chapter 5 which looks at all the relevant research on mite reduction.

Chapter 4

TREATMENT

As you might have gathered so far, the mite has cornered the market in survival and reproduction. We might not have noticed it quite as much if our bodies hadn't decided to develop antibodies to its faecal contents. Unfortunately, the tiniest airborne electrostatically charged particle of feacal droppings is enough to set off the allergic process and so it is not surprising that, in spite of all measures at reducing mite numbers, symptoms may persist. Fortunately, modern medicine has provided treatments which will reduce the allergic/inflammatory response and make life a bit more bearable for those afflicted.

The allergic manifestations may include asthma, rhinitis (nasal allergy), allergic conjunctivitis, contact dermatitis and eczema.

Asthmatics may react to many different physical and allergic stimuli but the mite is high on the list of potential allergens. The mainstay of treatment aims at reducing the chronic inflammation of the airways that results from those mast cells that have been stimulated to release histamine. The treatment is also directed at the white blood cells called eosinophils and others called T lymphocytes that are activated by allergy and enhance the inflammatory response. Corticosteroids suppress this reaction and asthmatics now have a choice of very effective corticosteroids that they can inhale directly to the site of the problem. The method of delivery to the lungs via inhaler devices has become much more efficient as treatment has evolved.

The allergic reaction is the same whether the mite allergen presents to the lungs, nose, eyes or skin and so corticosteroid preparations have been developed to address the site of allergic response. There are sprays and drops that will blanket the lining of the nasal passages and drops that can be instilled on to the conjunctivae of the eyes. There are ointments, lotions and creams that can be applied to the affected skin (provided it hasn't been secondarily infected by bacteria).

All of these corticosteroid preparations aim to treat with the least possible side effects. Absorption of corticosteroids into the blood stream in high enough quantities may result in systemic (general body) effects that could include bone thinning, diabetes, cataracts or even reduction in the manufacture of one's own natural steroids produced by the adrenal glands.

However, modern delivery systems, dosage and types of corticosteroid have helped to reduce such risks to much lower levels. Topical steroids for the skin may also be absorbed into the blood stream but use of the lower strength, intermittent, but still effective preparations has reduced such risks to a minimum.

Ultimately, in the most severe allergic responses, it may be necessary to treat with high doses of oral or intravenous corticosteroids, antihistamines and when life threatening, adrenaline may be required.

Antihistamines in the form of tablets (long acting and non-sedating) can act in conjunction with corticosteroids. They block the effects of released histamine. Other drugs, such as 'mast cell stabilisers' inhibit the release of histamine from mast cells and others act by reducing prostaglandin production. This suppresses another pathway of inflammation.

Another arm of treatment in the overall aim of controlling allergic symptoms has been the development of Leukotriene Receptor Antagonists (LTRAs). These work by blocking the effects of Leukotrienes which are released along with histamine and prostaglandins in the initial phases of the allergic reaction. Leukotrienes trigger contraction of smooth muscles lining the airways and small blood vessels. This can enhance the spasm of bronchi and increase the leakiness of blood vessels causing more mucous and, by attracting inflammatory white blood cells, increase local inflammation.

Such a wealth of options for treatment can be confusing and so the medical experts in this field have produced regular updates of guidelines so that patients and their doctors can collaborate on their management plans. The British Thoracic Society in collaboration with the Scottish Intercollegiate Guidelines Network have produced an update on asthma management in October 2014.

www.brit-thoracic.org.uk/document-library/clinical-information/asthma/btssign-asthma-guideline-2014/

The modern treatment of allergic manifestations has revolutionised the management of asthma, rhinitis, conjunctivitis and skin allergy. These treatments help to improve the quality of life of those who have a strong allergic response to the mite in spite of all efforts to reduce their cohabitation.

Chapter 5

RESEARCH

What is the evidence that reducing the numbers of mites will result in an improvement of associated symptoms?

The difficulty in answering this question arises from a number of issues.

- Individuals who are proven to be allergic to mites are often also allergic to a number of other allergens such as pollens and fur. Although there might be a successful reduction in the number of mites, symptoms may persist due to reactions to other allergens thus making it difficult to interpret any benefit.

- The studies that have attempted to answer this are of very variable quality. Some lack the necessary number of cases to prove any significant benefit.

- The baseline concentration of mites in the domestic environment will be different in the individual studies and the study subjects may be exposed to mites outside the domestic environment. In fact, research by Tovey ER et al [4] goes as far as to suggest, on the basis of personal sampling of subjects, that the greatest exposure occurred during the day and was associated with being active in domestic and crowded public situations. This may represent greater airborne exposure to allergen and endotoxin when compared with more settled allergen that would be expected in the bed situation. Compared with the average overall 24 hour exposure, the levels were actually lower in bed overnight. At the time of writing I am not aware as to whether this has been confirmed in any further studies.

- There may be differences in benefit depending on the allergic manifestation, whether this be asthma, rhinitis, eczema or conjunctivitis.

- There may be differences in response to reduction measures between children and adults.

- There is always the risk that subjects in such studies may take their medication more consistently once they are included in a trial and as a result appear to have benefited.

For all of these reasons and in spite of many such studies it has been difficult to come to any clear conclusion as to whether mite reduction offers significant health benefit in sensitized subjects.

The following are examples of some of the more recent research that has attempted to answer this question.

In the Cochrane review 19/01/15 authored by Nankervis H et al [5] they looked critically at the evidence from a number of studies as to whether mite reduction could reduce the severity of mite-associated **eczema**. They found 7 randomised controlled trials. These studies all include a placebo group in which e.g. no reduction measures or cotton bed covers (which would be ineffective), are used. There was a mixture of children and adult subjects and a variety of measures used to reduce mite numbers. They did not find any evidence to 'inform clinical practice'. There was no evidence of benefit in 6 studies and just a small benefit in one.

In another Cochrane review [6] of 55 randomised trials (3121 subjects), authored by Gotzsche PC and Johansen HK 16/04/08, they looked to see if there was any convincing evidence of benefit from mite reduction in **asthmatics** with mite allergy. Ten of the studies involved chemical methods of controlling mites, 37 used physical methods (26 included mattress encasing) and 8 used both. Many were considered poor trials and there was no difference in peak flow (measure of airflow in the airways), symptoms or need for medication.

The third Cochrane review of the literature authored by Sheikh A et al [7] in 07/07/10 looked at whether mite reduction would be of benefit in mite sensitive subjects with symptoms of **allergic rhinitis**. In summary, they concluded that acaracides (mite killing chemical) and extensive bedroom-based environmental control may be of some benefit in reducing rhinitis symptoms.

A review of research in the USA authored by Arroyave et al [8] in the Annals of Allergy, Asthma and Immunology 30/01/2014, concluded that use of expensive mattress covers made no difference to allergy symptoms in mite sensitive subjects. This was based on a critical appraisal of 24 studies.

This was in spite of the fact that they demonstrated a large effect in reducing mite population (around 20%). Unfortunately, however, this resulted in no statistically significant reduction in asthma, rhinitis or dermatitis. They speculated that perhaps the measures used don't reduce the mite population enough or that concentrating on the bedroom exposure isn't enough to produce benefit. Perhaps the exposure in public places is just as high (see research [4] quoted above).

There are other specialists in this field that would still recommend all the measures described above to reduce mite population as part of a comprehensive approach comprising allergen avoidance, effective medication and possibly immunotherapy.

What is the current evidence of effectiveness of immunotherapy in mite sensitive subjects?

Immunotherapy involves repeated injections of (initially) very small amounts of allergen under the skin (subcutaneous) followed by a gradual increase in the concentration of allergen injected at each visit. To demonstrate a reduction in allergic response that is lasting, may take 3 – 5 years of injections. An alternative method, currently being researched, is to present the allergen in a soluble tablet form, under the tongue.

A review of research in this field by Eifan AO et al [9] concluded that the majority of the studies at that time had involved small numbers of patients and variable doses of allergen. The studies were considered to be of variable quality. They confirmed that, provided there was careful patient selection, there was good evidence to support the efficacy of the subcutaneous approach to mite desensitization and its safety and long term benefit in adults and children. However, at that time, the evidence for a sublingual (under the tongue) approach was 'unconvincing' particularly in children. Studies are currently underway to determine the safe dose of sublingual allergen in selected mite sensitive subjects and more research is needed to determine its effectiveness both in the short and longer term when compared with subcutaneous immunotherapy.

Another potentially exciting development is the use of T cell epitopes instead of the full protein allergens in immunotherapy. Allergens are strips of protein made up of amino acids and epitopes are smaller sections of those protein strips (15 - 20 amino acids in length). Careful research has determined, for specific allergens, that identified small sections of their protein strips will serve just as well as the full allergen in the process of immunotherapy. The added advantage being that these epitopes are too small to cross link with antibodies on mast cells and trigger the release of histamine. This reduces the risk of allergic reactions occurring as a side effect of the immunotherapy.

Studies so far suggest that this approach to treatment is effective with few side effects for cat, grass pollen and house dust mite. The other advantage is the course of treatment is much shorter (4 injections into the skin) than current conventional subcutaneous immunotherapy which can be anything from 3 -5 years in duration.

Further trials are in the pipeline and it is hoped that these will confirm the optimism that is currently being expressed in the literature. A helpful summary of the current position can be found (for those with a background in allergology) in the State of the Art Review [10] in Clinical & Experimental Allergy of June 2015.

Do ionisers offer any benefit?

The most quoted study on the effect of ionisers on mite related symptoms by Warner J A et al [11] is the double blind, cross-over, placebo controlled study of 20 children with allergic asthma and mite allergy. They did confirm that ionisers produce a significant reduction of airborne concentration of mite allergen but there was a disappointing lack of any significant improvement in peak flow, symptom scores or need for treatment. They concluded that, although there was a significant reduction in mite allergen, there wasn't enough evidence to recommend ionisers as an effective management approach in mite related asthma. They didn't rule out their use as part of an integral more complex allergen avoidance regime.

Do air filtering systems offer any benefit?

Sublett J L [3] reviewed the effectiveness of air filters and cleaners in allergic respiratory disease. The point was made that when considering the benefits of air filtration there have been no clinical comparisons between the benefits of whole house filtration as opposed to portable room air cleaners. Poorly maintained whole house systems (e.g. forgetting to change the filter) may actually increase allergic symptoms. The meta-analysis of the only 10 randomised controlled trials on air filtration by McDonald E et al [12] did not reveal any differences in medication use, nasal symptoms or morning peak flow results.

Eight of the studies used sham filters as the placebo arm. There were some small significant improvements in total symptoms and sleep disturbance. Several of the studies reviewed looked at specific allergen reduction other than house dust mite. One study by Stillerman A et al [13] looked at the use of a localized air filtration system connected to a pillow encasement in a randomized controlled trial. The subjects (35) suffered from allergic nose and eye symptoms and were dog, cat or dust mite sensitive. There were significant improvements in nocturnal nasal and eye allergic symptoms and quality of life measures.

Conclusion

It is certainly possible that a comprehensive approach to mite reduction using acaracides, effective air filtration methods, pillow and mattress encasement along with all the other theoretical ways of impairing the mites existence, could result in a reduction in related allergic symptoms. However, the evidence that such intensive time consuming and, in some cases, costly measures are of proven value requires an equally comprehensive research protocol with large numbers of sufferers in a randomized, placebo controlled trial. This may be a challenge too far.

Fortunately not all humans are allergic to mites and although around 20 - 25% may have a positive skin test that doesn't mean that they will all have symptoms. It is probable that around half of those will be sufferers but that is a very large section of the population around the world and a significant burden for those with perennial symptoms.

Unfortunately, this book doesn't offer any magic bullet to counter this condition but it is hoped that it clarifies the scale and challenge that house dust mite allergy presents. Perhaps immunotherapy will be a more widely acceptable/affordable approach for those at the moderate to severe end of the spectrum and further research into its safety and methods of delivery are eagerly anticipated especially in the field of epitope peptides.

Even if a reduction in house dust mite population combined with effective immunotherapy were to significantly reduce mite allergy in an individual, there still remains the possibility that that individual may have more than one allergy and so may still suffer regular symptoms. Fortunately we have well tried and tested and effective treatments to counter these symptoms and improve quality of life.

HOUSE DUST MITE

OVERVIEW SUMMARY

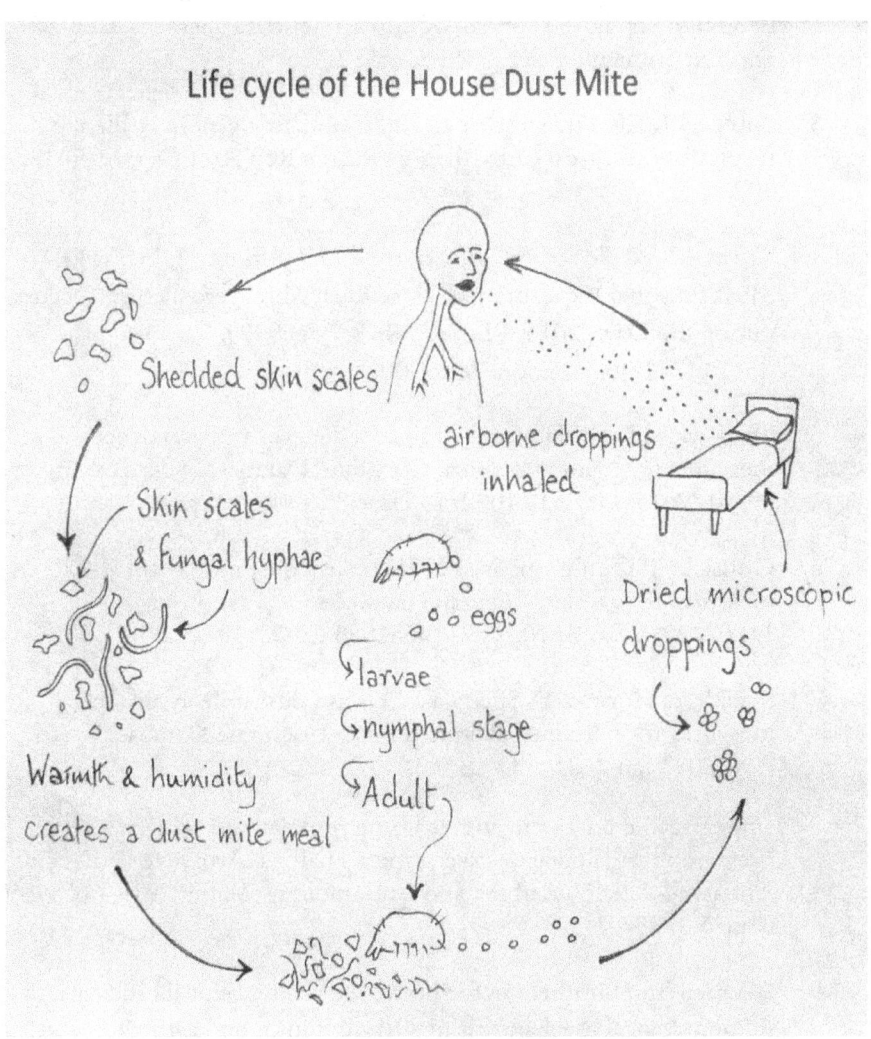

REFERENCES

1. Is Permanent Parasitism Reversible?—Critical Evidence from Early Evolution of House Dust Mites. Klimov P B & O'Connor B Systematic Biology p 1-13 2013

2. Custovic A, Taggart SCO, Kennaugh JH, Woodcock A. Portable dehumidifiers in the control of house dust mite allergens. Clinical and Experimental Allergy 1995;25:312-316

3. Sublett J L Effectiveness of air filters and air cleaners in allergic respiratory diseases. Curr Allergy Asthma Rep 2011 Oct; 11(5):395-402

4. Tovey ER, Willenborg CM, Crisafulli DA, Rimmer J, Marks GB Most Personal Exposure to House Dust Mite Aeroallergen Occurs during the Day. (2013) PLoS ONE 8(7): e69900. doi:10.1371/journal.pone.0069900

5. Nankervis H et al House dust mite reduction and avoidance measures for treating eczema. Cochrane Database (Skin Group) 19/01/2015. DOI: 10.1002/14651858.CD008426.pub2

6. Gotzsche P C and Johansen H K. House dust mite control measures for asthma Cochrane database (airways group). 11/07/2011. DOI: 10.1002/14651858.CD001187.pub3

7. Sheikh A, Hurwitz B, Shehata Y. House dust mite avoidance measures for perennial allergic rhinitis. Cochrane Database Syst Rev. 2007 Jan 24;(1):CD001563.

8. Impermeable dust mite covers in the primary and tertiary prevention of allergic disease: a meta-analysis. Arroyave W D et al. Annals of Allergy, Asthma and Immunology. March 2014 Vol 112, issue 3, p 237-248.

9. Allergen immunotherapy for house dust mite: clinical efficacy and immunological mechanisms in allergic rhinitis and asthma.
   Eifan AO, Calderon MA, Durham SR. Expert Opin Biol Ther. 2013 Nov;13(11):1543-56.

10 Immunoregulatory T cell epitope peptides: the new frontier in allergy therapy. Prickett S R, Rolland J M and O'Heir R E. Clinical & Experimental Allergy, vol 45, Issue 6, June 2015 p 1015-1026.

11 Double blind trial of ionisers in children with asthma sensitive to the house dust mite. Warner J A, Marchant J L, Warner J O. Thorax 1993;48:330-333.

12 Effect of air filtration systems on asthma: A systematic review of randomized trials. McDonald E et al. Chest 2 2002;122(5):1535-1542.

13 Efficacy of a novel air filtration pillow for avoidance of perennial allergens in symptomatic adults. Stillerman A et al Ann Allergy Asthma Immunol. 2010 May;104(5):440-9.

ABOUT THE AUTHOR

Dr Connellan is a retired Consultant Respiratory Physician who trained at St Mary's Hospital in London. His 35 years as a doctor provided a wealth of firsthand experience in all aspects of acute general and respiratory medicine. One of his specialist interests was the field of allergy and he investigated and treated a wide range of such cases over a 20 year period. These included allergies to food, drugs, insects and all the common airborne allergens. This has provided the stimulus, in his retirement, to provide short overviews of common allergic conditions without a lot of medical jargon, in simple and hopefully clear terms. He now lives with his wife in New Zealand in order to be closer to his children, grandchildren and extended family.

Other publications:

"The Medical Tactician: A Century of Doctor-Patient Relationships"
(ISBN 1468163469)

Dr Connellan takes readers back and forth between 1910 and present time for a comparison of doctor-patient relationships and medical practice. He juxtaposes his personal experiences as a modern day doctor with a compilation of articles from a medical practitioner working in London over a century ago.

"Hives & Skin Swelling ~ A Simple Guide"
(ISBN 147743934X)

This simple guide addresses the complex issues of acute and chronic urticaria/angio-oedema and their management. The cases are illustrated with simple graphics and individual case histories.

Printed by CreateSpace Independent Publishing Platform

www.ingramcontent.com/pod-product-compliance
Lightning Source LLC
Chambersburg PA
CBHW070733180526
45167CB00004B/1739